Mediterranean Diet Recipes & Cookbook

50 Mediterranean Diet Recipes + Our Free Mediterranean Diet Summary

M. Smith & R. King

Mediterranean Diet Recipes & Cookbook

Copyright © 2011 by M. Smith & R. King

"You must begin to think of yourself as becoming the person you want to be", **David Viscott**

Table of Contents

Mediterranean Diet Summary

The Mediterranean diet is a healthy eating diet that merges together different Mediterranean styles of cooking and healthy lifestyle benefits. All of this is brought together in a simple eating plan that many have adopted today for normal everyday eating.

Scientists have known about the healthy eating ideas of the Mediterranean since the mid 20th century. It wasn't until the early 1990's that it began to have an effect in the United States. Dr. Ansel Keys brought the knowledge of the Mediterranean diet to the US After recognizing its effects while stationed in Italy. Oldways and the Harvard School of Pubic Health introduced this style of eating during a conference in 1993. They introduced the Mediterranean Diet Pyramid to Americans. The pyramid made it easy to understand how the diet works and opened up a new phase for a healthier way of eating. Recognized as the "gold standard", this diet is a pattern for a lifetime of healthy eating.

There are two approaches to nutrition in Western Europe. The first approach is the northern European way of eating, which is followed by most of the United States as well as

Austria, Germany, Switzerland and Belgium. These diets include large quantities of red meat, butter and animal fats. It also includes low amounts of fresh fruits and vegetables. This is not considered a very healthy way of eating and contributes to heart disease, high cholesterol and numerous other life threatening diseases.

The southern European approach is the Mediterranean diet. Places such as southern France, Italy, Spain and Greece, countries that boarder on the Mediterranean coast include large quantities of fresh fruits and vegetables, Their fat intake is low and consists of good fats such as monounsaturated and polyunsaturated fats. This factor has lead to the belief that this diet has significantly lowered the risks of obesity, diabetes, cancer, cardiovascular disease and other health related problems in these southern European countries.

Many studies show that adopting the Mediterranean diet into eating habits leads to a longer life expectancy than those who follow the northern European way of eating. There are many factors of the Mediterranean diet that can lead us to better health. The use of olive oil instead of oils that are rich in saturated fats can lower blood sugar levels, cholesterol levels and blood pressure levels. Eating lower quantities of processed foods and eating higher levels of fresh foods and fish are all factors of the Mediterranean diet.

There are many studies comparing different diets to ones health. Studies show that people who have adopted the Mediterranean way of eating have a lower risk of developing high blood pressure and high cholesterol as well as the other heart related problems. It has also been shown that following this diet reduces the risk of life threatening diseases such as cancer, diabetes, Alzheimer's and Parkinson's disease.

There are a number of healthy components to this diet. As with most diets it encourages getting plenty of exercise. Exercise is very important when it comes to maintaining a healthy body no matter what type of eating habits we are used to. It gets the blood flowing as well as adding to energy levels and aides against obesity.

When it comes to the food ingested the Mediterranean diets looks at the food components a little differently than most other diets plans. One of the main factors is replacing fats, such as butter, with olive or canola oil. Olive oil is a monounsaturated fat that helps to lower cholesterol as well as providing our bodies with antioxidants. Canola oil is a polyunsaturated fat that contains Omega-3. This fatty acid helps to lower the risk of sudden heart attacks, helps to moderate blood pressure, decreases the clotting of blood and lowers triglycerides. Fatty fish such as trout, tuna, salmon and mackerel all contain Omega-3 fatty acids.

Eating fish and poultry at least two times a week is another factor of the Mediterranean diet. Fatty fish filled with Omega-3 are healthy choices. Grilling or baking fish makes it an even healthier choice. Fried fish should only be eaten if cooked in low amounts of canola or olive oil.

Red meat isn't completely removed but should be limited to only a couple of times a month. Substitute chicken, turkey or fish for steaks and burgers. If red meats are included be sure they are lean cuts of meat and in small amounts. It's best to avoid high fat meats such as bacon and sausage all together.

Fresh fruits and vegetables are high on the diet. Some countries such as Greece include up to nine servings a day. It is suggested that between seven and nine servings should be included in the daily diet. Studies have shown that choosing fruits and vegetables over other fatty or processed foods can lower bad cholesterol and decrease the risk of fatty deposit buildups in the arteries and veins.

Whole grains are included in the Mediterranean diet. Whole grains found in pasta, rice and bread contain very tiny amounts of trans fat. Trans fats can lead high blood pressure and heart attacks. When eating bread don't use butter. Try dipping your bread in olive oil, even flavored olive oil or just eat it plain.

Nuts which include pistachio and cashews, although high in fat are still considered healthy in small amounts. Eighty percent of the calories in nuts come from fat but it's not saturated fat. A handful of nuts a day as a quick snack can be a benefit to ones health. Try to avoid nuts that are heavily salted, honey roasted or candy coated.

It's also best to shy away from using an over abundance of salt on foods. Herbs and spices can be substituted when seasoning foods. Fresh herbs and spices are a much healthier choice and give foods a wonderful taste and aroma.

Incorporating low fat cheese, skim milk and fat free yogurt into a healthy eating plan is also a factor of the Mediterranean diet. These are great alternatives for ice cream, whole or two percent milk and most types of cheese, which are high in unhealthy fat content.

A small amount of red wine is also included in the Mediterranean diet. In moderation red wine has been contributed in lowering the risk of heart disease. Women should limit their intake to about 5 ounces a day. Men under 65 should only consume about 10 ounces a day and men over 65 should stay at the 5 ounce or below mark.

The use of alcohol and its effect on our health has always been a pondered issue. Many have their doubts about incorporating it into their daily diets. If there's a family history of liver disease, migraine headaches or alcohol abuse or if you don't normally drink alcohol substitute grape juice. If you're not an alcohol drinker be sure to consult with your doctor before adding it to your diet regime.

To put it all in perspective, adopting the Mediterranean diet has been proven to prevent major chronic diseases which leads to a longer and healthier life. This is the reason why most scientific institutes encourage people to follow the guidelines of the Mediterranean diet. It's a nutritious as well as a delicious way to achieve a healthier lifestyle. Eating foods low in fat, full of antioxidants and other health promoting substances has proven to extend life and decrease the risk of disease. Many people who have switched to the Mediterranean diet say they will never go back to eating any other way. If a healthy life is what you're looking for, it might pay to take a look at this diet and enjoy some of the healthier foods it has to offer.

Banana Berry Beverage

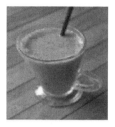

Ingredients:

1/2 C frozen cranberries

1 ripe banana, sliced

1 C vanilla rice milk

1 splash cranberry juice

1 tbsp vanilla protein powder

Directions:

Place the cranberries and banana into the blender.

Add the milk and cranberry juice.

Top with the protein powder.

Cover the blender and blend until smooth and frothy.

Dairy Free Strawberry Smoothie

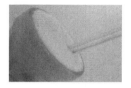

Ingredients:

1 C of cold vanilla hemp milk

1 C chilled strawberries, sliced

1 tsp honey

Directions:

Pour the hemp milk into the blender.

Add the strawberries and honey.

Blend until smooth and creamy.

Yogurt and Honey Breakfast Fruit

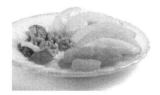

Ingredients:

1 apricot, halved and pitted

1 small pear, peeled and sliced

4 tbsp plain non fat yogurt

1 tbsp honey

1 tbsp walnuts, chopped

Directions:

Place the apricots and pear slices onto a plate.

In a bowl whisk together the yogurt and honey.

Fold in the walnuts.

Use as a dip or top the fruit with a spoonful.

Feta Garlic Sausage Patties

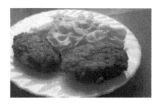

Ingredients:

1 1/2 lbs ground lamb

1 garlic clove, pressed

1 1/2 tsp kosher salt

1/3 C feta cheese, finely crumbled

1 tbsp fresh mint, chopped fine

1 tbsp extra virgin olive oil

Directions:

Crumble the lamb into a mixing bowl.

Add the garlic and salt and mix until well blended.

Using your hands form the lamb mixture into balls.

Use your finger and make an indention in each of the balls.

Fill the indention with a little cheese and mint.

Reform the meat into a ball around the filling.

Flatten each ball into a patty.

Place the oil into a skillet and place the skillet over medium high heat.

Add the sausage patties and cook 3 minutes or until brown on the bottom.

Turn the patties and cook an additional 3 minutes or until cooked through.

Herbed Vegetable Omelet

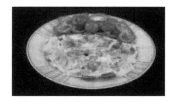

Ingredients:

1 tomato, diced

1 green bell pepper, diced

1/4 C black olives, pitted and diced

1 garlic clove, minced

2 green onions, chopped

1 tsp olive oil

1 tsp lemon juice

4 eggs

2 tbsp skim milk

1 tsp dried chives

1 tsp dried basil

1 tsp dried oregano

2 oz feta cheese, crumbled

Directions:

Place the tomatoes, bell pepper, olives, garlic and green onions in a bowl.

In a separate bowl whisk together the oil and lemon juice.

Pour the mixture over the vegetables and toss to coat.

Let stand for a few minutes for the vegetables to absorb the flavor.

Place the eggs and milk in a separate bowl.

Add the chives, basil and oregano and whisk until well blended.

Heat a non stick skillet over medium heat.

Pour half of the egg mixture into the pan and cook 2 minutes or until beginning to brown.

Add half of the vegetable mixture onto one side of the omelet.

Sprinkle the vegetables with half of the cheese.

Shrimp and Zucchini Omelet

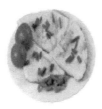

Ingredients:

3 tbsp extra virgin olive oil, divided

1/4 C onion, chopped

1 zucchini, peeled and chopped

1 tomato, chopped

1 C small shrimp, cooked

10 eggs, whisked

1/2 tsp salt

1/4 tsp pepper

Directions:

Pour 1 tbsp of the oil into a large skillet and place over medium heat/

Sir the onions into the oil and cook 3 minutes or until just tender.

Stir the zucchini into the onions and continue to cook 10 minutes, stirring occasionally or until the zucchini is fork tender.

Transfer the vegetables to a sieve and drain well then place in mixing bowl.

Add the tomatoes and shrimp and toss to combine.

Pour the eggs into the bowl and sprinkle with the salt and pepper.

Pour the remaining oil into the skillet and place over high heat.

Pour the egg vegetable mixtures into the hot oil and cook 5 minutes or until the eggs are set.

When the eggs are set fold the egg mixture in half and cook 2 additional minutes or until cooked through.

Arugula Tomato and Red Onion Salad

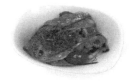

Ingredients:

3 tbsp olive oil, divided

2 C stale whole wheat bread, cubed

1 C cherry tomatoes cut in half

8 C arugula, torn

1/4 C red onion, cut into rings

1 tbsp garlic, minced

1/4 tsp salt

1/8 tsp pepper

2 tbsp red wine vinegar

1/2 Parmesan cheese, grated

Directions:

Pour half of the oil into a skillet and place over medium high heat.

Add the bread cubes and stirring occasionally brown for 5 minutes or until just crispy.

Add the tomatoes, arugula and onion and stirring constantly cook 1 minute or just until the arugula begins to wilt.

Push all the ingredients to the back side of the skillet.

Pour the remaining oil into the skillet.

Add the garlic and stirring constantly cook for 30 seconds or until fragrant.

Stir the garlic and the remaining salad mixture together in the skillet.

Remove the skillet from the stove and stir in the salt and pepper.

Pour the vinegar over the salad and stir to coat well.

Place in a serving bowl and sprinkle the cheese over the top.

Couscous Tomato and Cucumber Salad

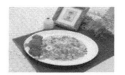

Ingredients:

1 C of water

2 tsp olive oil

1/2 C whole wheat couscous

1 cucumber, peeled and chopped

1 tomato, chopped

1/2 C feta cheese, crumbled

1 tsp dried dill

2 tbsp lemon juice

Directions:

Place the water and olive oil into a saucepan, place over high heat and bring to a boil.

Stir in the couscous and bring back to a brisk boil.

Reduce the heat to low, cover the pan and simmer for 2 minutes.

Remove the pan from the heat, leave covered and let stand 5 minutes.

Fluff the couscous with a fork.

Place the cucumbers, tomatoes and cheese into a bowl and toss gently.

Stir in the couscous and sprinkle with the dill.

Pour the lemon juice into the bowl and gently stir to coat well.

Vegetable and Black Olive Salad

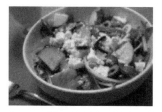

Ingredients:

1/3 C red wine vinegar

2 tbsp extra virgin olive oil

1 tsp dried dill

1 tsp garlic powder

1/4 tsp salt

1/4 tsp pepper

6 cups lettuce, chopped

2 tomatoes, quartered

1 cucumber, peeled and sliced

1 red onion, sliced thin

1/2 C ripe black olives, sliced

1/2 C feta cheese, crumbled

Directions:

Pour the vinegar and olive oil into a bowl.

Add the dill, garlic powder, salt and pepper and whisk until well blended.

Place the lettuce into a salad bowl.

Add the tomatoes, cucumbers and onion tossing to combine with the lettuce.

Spread the sliced olives over the top of the salad.

Pour the dressing over the salad and gently toss to coat.

Sprinkle with the cheese just before serving.

Grilled Shrimp and Lime Salad

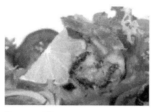

Ingredients:

3/4 C extra virgin olive oil

1 tbsp lime juice

1/4 C red wine vinegar

1 tsp Dijon mustard

2 tsp garlic, minced

1 lb large shrimp, deveined

1 (16 oz) pkg salad mix

2 large tomatoes, quartered

1 lime, sliced thin

Directions:

Pour the oil, lime juice and vinegar into a bowl.

Add the Dijon mustard and garlic and whisk until well combined.

Remove half of the marinade to another bowl and set aside.

Place the shrimp in the remaining marinade and let stand 30 minutes.

Heat the grill.

Thread the shrimp onto metal skewers.

Grill, turning occasionally, for 8 minutes or until cooked through.

Place the salad mix into a bowl.

Spread the shrimp, tomatoes and lime slices over the top of the salad.

Parsley Veggie Salad

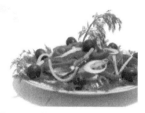

Ingredients:

1/4 C fresh parsley, chopped

1 cucumber, sliced thin

2 red sweet peppers, seeds removed and sliced

1 red onion, sliced thin

1/4 C black olives, pitted and sliced

2 tbsp extra virgin olive oil

1 tbsp white wine vinegar

1/4 tsp salt

1/8 tsp pepper

Directions:

Place the parsley in the bottom of a salad bowl.

Layer the cucumbers, peppers, onions and olives over the parsley.

In a bowl whisk together the oil, vinegar, salt and pepper until blended well.

Pour the dressing over the salad just before serving.

Mint and Bulgur Salad

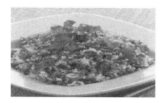

Ingredients:

1 C of water

1/2 C bulgur

1/4 C of lemon juice

1 tbsp extra virgin olive oil

1/2 tsp garlic, minced

1/4 tsp salt

1/8 tsp pepper

2 C flat leaf parsley, chopped very fine

1/4 C fresh mint, chopped

2 tomatoes, diced

1 cucumber, peeled, seeds removed and diced

4 scallions, sliced very thin

Directions:

Place the water into a small saucepan.

Add the bulgur and bring to a boil.

Remove the pan from the heat and cover.

Let stand 25 minutes or until most of the water is absorbed and the bulgur is soft.

If any water remains drains through a small sieve.

Place the bulgur into a large bowl and let cool.

Pour the lemon juice and oil into a small bowl.

Whisk in the garlic, salt and pepper until blended well.

When the bulgur has cooled add he parsley, mint, tomatoes, cucumber and scallions.

Pour the dressing over the top and toss to coat.

Grilled Lamb Dinner Salad

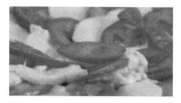

Ingredients:

1 lb boneless lamb steak

1 1/2 tsp salt, divided

1/4 tsp pepper

2 cucumbers, sliced thin

1 tomato, sliced thin

1/2 C red onions, minced

1/4 C feta cheese

1/4 fresh mint leaves

1/4 C lemon juice

1 tsp extra virgin olive oil

Directions:

Heat the grill to high.

Sprinkle both sides of the lamb steak 1/2 tsp of salt and the pepper.

Place the lamb on the heat grill and cook for 4 minutes.

Turn and cook an additional 4 minutes or until cooked the desired doneness.

Remove the steak and set aside.

Place the cucumbers, tomato, onion, cheese and mint leaves into a bowl.

In a small bowl whisk together the lemon juice and oil. Pour the mixture over the salad.

Slice the lamb steak into thin strips then cut the strips into bite size pieces.

Add the lamb to the salad and toss to combine well.

Tuna and Veggie Salad

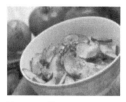

Ingredients:

1 tsp salt

Juice from 1 lemon

1 lb radishes, grated

2 tbsp fresh parsley, minced

1/4 C celery, diced small

1/4 C scallions, minced

2 tomatoes, quartered

3 tbsp olive oil

1 (3.75 oz) can of tuna in water, drained and chunked

Salad greens

Directions:

Place the salt and lemon juice into a bowl and whisk to combine.

Add the radishes, parsley, celery and scallions and stir to coat well.

Let the mixture stand for 5 minutes.

Drain the mixture well and place in a salad bowl.

Add the tomatoes to the salad and drizzle the salad with oil, tossing to coat.

Add the tuna and toss again to combine.

Serve over a bed of crisp salad greens.

Fresh Spinach and Red Pepper Salad

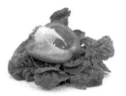

Ingredients:

1 lb. fresh spinach leaves, torn

1 C sweet red bell pepper, chopped

1 C fresh mushrooms, sliced

1 garlic clove, minced

2 tbsp olive oil

1 tbsp red wine vinegar

1 1/2 tsp mustard

1/4 tsp salt

1/8 tsp pepper

Directions:

Place the spinach, bell peppers and mushrooms into a salad bowl and toss.

Place the garlic into a mixing bowl.

Add the oil, vinegar, mustard, salt and pepper and whisk until blended together well.

Pour the dressing over the salad and toss to coat well.

Monkfish Soup with Pasta

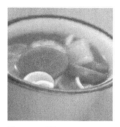

Ingredients:

2 tbsp olive oil

1 onion, chopped

1 tbsp garlic, minced

4 C of water

1 carrot, sliced

1 (6 oz) can tomatoes, diced small

1 C of rotini pasta, uncooked

1/4 tsp dried rosemary

1/2 tsp salt

1/4 tsp pepper

1 lb monkfish, cut into bite size pieces

Directions:

Pour the oil into a sauce pan and place over medium high heat.

Stir in the onion and garlic and stirring often, cook 5 minutes or until tender.

Pour the water into the pan.

Stir in the carrot, tomatoes and pasta.

Add the rosemary, salt and pepper and stir to combine.

Bring to a brisk boil then reduce the heat medium.

Simmer for 20 minutes or until the carrots are tender.

Stir in the fish pieces.

Simmer the soup for 10 minutes longer or until the fish is cooked through.

Lentil Broccoli and Carrot Soup

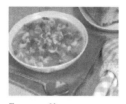

Ingredients:

2 tbsp olive oil

1 onion, chopped

2 carrots, peeled and chopped

1 tsp cumin

1 tsp fennel seed

8 C of water

1 1/2 C brown lentil

1 C broccoli florets

Juice from 1 lemon

Directions:

Pour the oil into a large kettle and place over medium high heat.

Stir in the onions and carrots.

Cook, stirring often, for 15 minutes or until the vegetables are tender.

Sprinkle the cumin and fennel seed over the vegetables and stir to combine.

Pour the water into the kettle.

Stir in the lentils.

Bring the soup to a boil.

Reduce the heat and simmer 20 minutes.

Add the broccoli and bring the soup back to a boil.

Reduce the heat and simmer 15 minutes or until the broccoli is tender.

Stir in the lemon juice just before serving.

Halibut Perch Soup

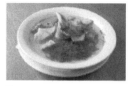

Ingredients:

1 C of extra virgin olive oil

2 garlic cloves, peeled

1 onion, chopped fine

2 tomatoes, chopped fine

1 lb potatoes cut into thin slices

2 C of fish stock

1 tsp salt

1 lb halibut fillets, cut into pieces

1 lb perch fillets, cut into pieces

2 sprigs of fresh parsley, chopped

4 almonds, toasted

Directions:

Pour the oil into a Dutch oven pan and place over high heat.

Stir in the garlic cloves and fry, stirring often, for 5 minutes or until golden brown.

Remove the garlic and set aside.

Add the onion to the pan and cook, stirring occasionally, for 4 minutes or until translucent.

Reduce the heat to medium low and stir in the tomatoes, cooking for 10 minutes.

Place the potatoes into the pan and pour in the fish stock.

Cook for 10 minutes then sprinkle in the salt.

Add the fish and adjust the heat to medium high.

Cook 15 minutes or until the potatoes are tender.

Be careful not to overcook the fish it should never cook longer than 20 minutes.

Mediterranean Chicken Stew

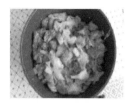

Ingredients:

2 tbsp + 2 tsp of extra virgin olive oil, divided

3 onions, chopped

2 garlic cloves, minced

1/2 C of flour

4 lb bone in chicken thighs, skin removed

1 tsp salt, divided

1/4 tsp pepper

1 C dry white wine

1/2 lb button mushrooms, quartered

4 plum tomatoes, chopped

2 carrots, chopped

1 C reduced sodium chicken broth

2 bay leaves

3/4 tsp dried rosemary

Directions:

Place 2 tsp of the oil into a Dutch oven or large saucepan and place over medium heat.

Add the onion and cook, stirring often, for 5 minutes.

Stir in the garlic and cook an additional 4 minutes or until the onion is soft.

Remove the pan from the heat and place the onions in a bowl, set aside.

Place the flour in a shallow dish.

Sprinkle the chicken with half of the salt and dredge through the flour coating well.

Place the remaining oil in the Dutch oven and add the chicken.

Cook the chicken over medium heat for 5 minutes per side or until nicely browned.

Remove the chicken and set aside.

Pour the wine into the Dutch oven and scraping any brown bits from the bottom of the pan, cook for 1 minute.

Stir in the mushrooms, tomatoes, carrot, broth bay leaves and rosemary.

Return the onions and chicken to the pan being sure the chicken is at least partially submerged in the liquid.

Bring the mixture to a boil, reduce the heat to low, partially cover the pan and cook 1 hour or until the chicken is very tender and cooked through.

Mediterranean Chicken Stew

Lightly Sauced Baked Salmon

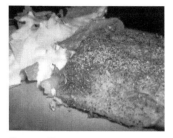

Ingredients:

8 oz salmon fillets

1 tsp olive oil

2 tbsp dry white wine

1 small onion, sliced thin

1 garlic clove, chopped fine

1 C tomatoes, diced

1/8 tsp orange zest, grated

1/8 tsp dried oregano

1/4 tsp salt, divided

1/4 tsp pepper, divided

Directions:

Set the oven temperature to 450 degrees and preheat.

Heat the oil in a skillet over high heat until hot but not smoking.

Stir the onion into the hot oil and cook, stirring often, for 4 minutes or until browned.

Stir the garlic into the onion and pour the wine into the skillet.

Simmer for 1 minute.

Stir in the tomatoes, orange zest, oregano and half of the salt and pepper.

Simmer for 3 minutes, stirring often.

Season the salmon with the remaining salt and pepper.

Place the salmon into a baking dish and pour the sauce over the salmon.

Bake the salmon, uncovered, for 15 minutes or just until the fish is cooked through.

Broiled Salmon with Veggies

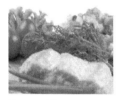

Ingredients:

1 lb salmon

1/2 lb tomatoes, chopped

2 C carrots, grated

1 zucchini, grated

1/4 C cilantro, chopped

3 tbsp olive oil

2 tbsp white wine vinegar

1/4 tsp salt

1/4 tsp pepper

Directions:

Preheat the broiler.

Place the salmon on a broiler pan.

Broil the salmon 4 minutes then turn.

Continue to broil 4 minutes or until the salmon flakes easily with a fork.

Remove and place on a platter.

Place the tomatoes, carrots, zucchini and cilantro into a bowl.

Whisk together the oil, vinegar, salt and pepper in a separate bowl

Pour the mixture over the vegetables and toss to coat.

Serve the vegetables over the salmon or on the side.

Baked Coconut Cod

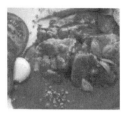

Ingredients:

4 cod fillets, cut into pieces

1/2 tsp salt

1 garlic clove, minced

3 tbsp cilantro, chopped

2 tbsp coconut, shredded

1/2 C tomato paste

Directions:

Set the oven to 350 degrees and preheat

Sprinkle the salt over the cod pieces.

In a bowl mix together the garlic, cilantro, coconut and tomato paste until well blended.

Press the coconut mixture into the pieces of cod.

Lay the cod pieces on a piece of foil and fold the foil around the cod closing tightly.

Place the foil wrapped cod into a baking dish.

Bake the cod for 25 minutes or until the cod is cooked through.

Broiled Raisin Trout

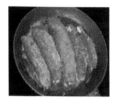

Ingredients:

6 trout fillets

1/2 C extra virgin olive oil

1/4 fresh lemon juice

1/4 tsp pepper

1 garlic clove, minced

1/2 C golden raisins

Broiled Raisin Trout

Directions:

Place the trout into a glass dish in a single layer.

In a bowl combine the oil, lemon juice and pepper.

Pour half of the mixture over the fish, turning to coat.

Cover and refrigerate for at least 1 hour.

Preheat the broiler.

Remove the fish and discard the marinade.

Place the fish on a broiler pan.

Broil 3 inches from the heat for 8 minutes, turning occasionally for even browning.

Remove, place on a platter and keep warm.

Place the reserved marinade into a saucepan.

Add the raisins and bring the mixture to a brisk boil.

Pour the sauce over the fish before serving.

Baked Halibut Steaks

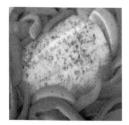

Ingredients:

2 tsp olive oil

1/2 tsp fennel seed, crushed

2 garlic cloves, sliced thin

1/4 C lemon juice

2 C of carrots, cut into thin strips

1 C green bell pepper, cut into thin strips

1 C zucchini, cut into thin strips

4 (6 oz) halibut steaks

Directions:

Set the oven temperature to 375 degrees and preheat.

Pour the oil into a skillet and place over medium high heat.

Stir in the fennel and garlic and cook, stirring constantly for 3 minutes.

Remove from the heat, cool slightly and stir in the lemon juice.

Cut four 15 inch squares of aluminum foil.

Place 1/4 of the vegetables onto each piece of foil.

Add a halibut stead to each packet and top each with 1/4 of the garlic mixture.

Fold and tightly seal the foil around the fish.

Place the packets on a baking sheet.

Bake 25 minutes or until the fish flakes easily with a fork and vegetables are tender.

Chicken and Walnut Green Beans

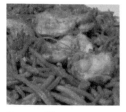

Ingredients:

1/2 C olive oil

1/3 C lemon juice

1 1/2 C cilantro

8 boneless, skinless chicken thighs

1 lb. fresh green beans, rinsed and trimmed

1 C of walnuts

3 tbsp walnut oil

1 garlic clove

1/2 tsp salt

1/4 tsp pepper

Directions:

Pour the olive oil and lemon juice into the blender.

Add the cilantro and blend until the cilantro is chopped fine.

Remove 1/2 C of the marinade and pour into a large bowl.

Place the chicken into the marinade turning to coat.

Cover the chill for at least 30 minutes.

Place the green beans into a pan and cover completely with water.

Place the pan over high heat and bring the water to a brisk boil.

Reduce the heat to medium and cook the beans 10 minutes or until tender.

Drain the beans, rinse with cold water and drain again.

Preheat the grill to medium high.

Remove the chicken from the marinade and place on the preheated grill.

Grill the chicken 20 minutes, turning often, or until the juices run clear.

Place the remaining marinade mixture back into the blender.

Three Pepper Chicken

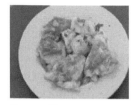

Ingredients:

8 skinless chicken thighs

1/2 tsp salt

1/4 tsp pepper

2 tbsp olive oil

1 sweet red bell pepper, cut into slices

1 sweet yellow bell pepper, cut into slices

1 green bell pepper, cut into slices

1 onion, sliced thin

1 garlic clove, minced

1 1/2 tsp Italian seasoning

2 tbsp balsamic vinegar

1 C tomatoes, crushed

Directions:

Coat the chicken evenly on both sides with the salt and pepper.

Place the oil into a skillet and place over medium high heat.

Add the chicken and cook 15 minutes, turning often, or until cooked through and browned.

Remove the chicken and keep warm.

Place the bell peppers and onion into the skillet.

Cook 3 minutes or until soft.

Stir in the garlic and Italian seasoning and stirring constantly cook 1 minute.

Pour in the vinegar and add the tomatoes stirring to combine.

Cook 4 minutes, stirring occasionally until heated through.

Pour the mixture over the chicken before serving.

Lemon Garlic Tofu

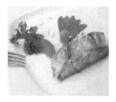

Ingredients:

1/4 C lemon juice

1 tbsp olive oil

3 garlic cloves, minced

1 tsp dried oregano

1/2 tsp salt

1/4 tsp pepper

14 oz extra firm water packed tofu

Directions:

Pour the lemon juice and olive oil into a small bowl.

Add the garlic, oregano, salt and pepper and whisk to combine.

Reserve 2 tbsp of the mixture.

Wash and pat dry the tofu.

Cut the tofu into 1/2 inch thick slices.

Place the sliced tofu into a shallow baking dish.

Pour the lemon juice mixture over the tofu and turn the tofu to coat evenly.

Let stand for 30 minutes.

Preheat the grill to medium high.

Lightly oil the grill rack.

Place the tofu on the prepared grill and cook 4 minutes, basting once with reserved mixture.

Turn, baste again and grill for 4 minutes longer or until the tofu is lightly browned.

Multi Colored Stuffed Peppers

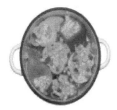

Ingredients:

5 tbsp olive oil, divided

1 lb ground pork

3 garlic cloves, chopped

3 sprigs fresh parsley, chopped fine

1/2 tsp nutmeg

1/2 tsp cinnamon,

1/4 tsp pepper

1/4 tsp oregano

4 tomatoes, peeled and chopped fine

1 1/2 tsp salt, divided

1 tsp sugar

1 1/4 C of water, divided

8 tbsp short grain rice, uncooked

2 red bell peppers

2 yellow bell peppers

Directions:

Place 4 tbsp of the oil into a Dutch oven placed over medium high heat.

Add the pork, garlic and parsley.

Sprinkle in the nutmeg, cinnamon, pepper and oregano.

Cook, stirring often for 8 minutes or until the pork is a golden brown.

Remove 2 tbsp of the chopped tomato and set aside.

Add the remaining tomato, 1 tsp salt and sugar and stir to blend in well.

Reduce the heat to medium low, cover the pan and cook 5 minutes or the tomatoes are very juicy.

Roasted Rosemary Portobello

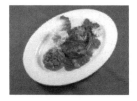

Ingredients:

1 lb Portobello mushrooms, washed and trimmed

1/4 C garlic flavored olive oil

1/4 tsp pepper

1/8 tsp sea salt

2 bunches of rosemary sprigs

Directions:

Set the oven to 425 degrees and preheat.

Place the mushrooms into a large bowl.

Pour the oil over the mushrooms and toss to coat.

Sprinkle with the salt and pepper.

Allow the mushrooms to stand in the mixture for 10 minutes.

Remove 1 rosemary sprig and set aside.

Arrange the remaining rosemary sprigs over the bottom of roasting pan.

Transfer the mushrooms to the pan laying them evenly over the rosemary.

Roast the mushrooms 15 minutes or until tender.

Chop the remaining rosemary sprig and sprinkle over the mushrooms before serving.

Green Beans and Tomatoes

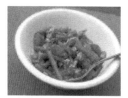

Ingredients:

3 1/4 lb fresh green beans, washed and trimmed

3 tomatoes, chopped coarsely

2 tbsp extra virgin olive oil

1 1/2 tbsp red wine vinegar

Directions:

Fill a saucepan 2/3 full of water and place over high heat.

Bring the water to a brisk boil.

Place the green beans in a steamer basket and place the basket over the boiling water.

Cover the basket and steam the green beans for 5 minutes or until tender.

Rinse the beans under cold water and drain well.

Place the beans into a serving bowl.

Add the tomatoes and toss gently to combine.

In a small bowl whisk the oil and vinegar together .

Pour the mixture over the beans and tomatoes and toss to coat.

Lemon Zucchini

Ingredients:

1 tbsp olive oil

1 lb zucchini, sliced into 1/2 inch pieces

1 1/2 tbsp parsley, chopped

1 tbsp lemon juice

1/4 tsp pepper

Directions:

Pour the oil into a skillet and place over medium heat.

Add the zucchini and cook 2 minutes stirring often.

Reduce the heat to low and cover the skillet.

Continue cooking 4 minutes or until the zucchini is tender.

Transfer the zucchini to a bowl.

Add the parsley, lemon juice and pepper and toss to coat.

Balsamic Spinach with Nuts

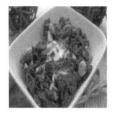

Ingredients:

2 tsp extra virgin olive oil

2 garlic cloves, minced

2 tbsp raisins

1 tbsp pine nuts

1 (10 oz) bag of fresh spinach

2 tsp balsamic vinegar

1/4 tsp salt

1/8 tsp pepper

1 tbsp Parmesan cheese, grated

Directions:

Pour the oil into a skillet and place over medium high heat.

Place the garlic, raisins and pine nuts into the skillet and stirring constantly cook 30 seconds or until fragrant.

Add the spinach and stirring constantly cook 3 minutes or just until the spinach is wilted.

Transfer the mixture to a serving bowl.

Pour the vinegar over the spinach, sprinkle with the salt and pepper and toss to coat well.

Top with the grated Parmesan cheese just before serving.

Cinnamon and Nut Topped Oranges

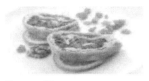

Ingredients:

1 tbsp sugar

1 tsp cinnamon

2 oranges cut in half

1/8 C walnuts, chopped

Cinnamon and Nut Topped Oranges

Directions:

Place the sugar into a small mixing bowl.

Add the cinnamon and stir until well combined.

Sprinkle the cinnamon sugar evenly over the oranges.

Top the oranges with chopped walnuts and serve.

Rose Apple Side Dish

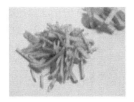

Ingredients:

3 sweet apples, peeled, seeds removed and sliced into sticks

2 tbsp sugar

2 tbsp lemon juice

1 tbsp rose water

1 dash of salt

Rose Apple Side Dish

Directions:

Place half of the apples into a blender

Sprinkle in the sugar.

Add the lemon juice and rose water.

Sprinkle in the salt

Cover the blender and blend 30 seconds or until coarsely chopped.

Add the remaining apples and blend another 20 seconds.

Pears in Pomegranate Sauce

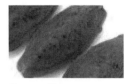

Ingredients:

4 ripe Bosc pears, quartered

1 1/2 C of pomegranate juice

1 C sweet dessert wine

Directions:

Place the pear quarters into a Dutch oven pan.

Pour the juice and wine over the pears and place the pan over medium high heat.

Bring the juice to a simmer then reduce the heat to low. Cover the pan and simmer 30 minutes, turning the pears over a couple of times during cooking.

Remove the pears with a slotted spoon and set aside.

Adjust the heat under the cooking juice to high.

Boil 10 minutes or until reduced to half.

Pour the juice over the pears before serving.

Herbed Rice and Brown Lentils

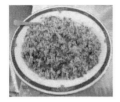

Ingredients:

1 C brown lentils, washed and drained

4 tbsp olive oil

1 C long grain rice

1 tbsp cumin

1 tsp salt

1/2 tsp turmeric

1/2 tsp pepper

1 1/2 C of warm water

Directions:

Place the lentils into a large saucepan and cover completely with water.

Place the saucepan over high heat and bring the water to a brisk boil.

Remove the pan from the heat, cover and let stand for 10 minutes.

Drain the lentils, rinse under cold water and drain again.

Pour the oil into a large pan and place over medium heat.

Stir the lentils and rice into the hot oil.

Stirring constantly cook for 2 minutes or until well coated.

Stir in the cumin, salt, turmeric and pepper well.

Pour the water into the pan and stirring constantly allow the water to come to a full boil.

Reduce the heat to low, cover the pan and cook 10 minutes or until all the water has evaporated.

Cornmeal Polenta

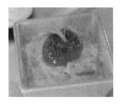

Ingredients:

6 C of cold water

1 1/3 C of cornmeal

1 tsp salt

Directions:

Pour the water into a saucepan and place the pan over medium high heat.

Stir in the cornmeal and salt and bring the mixture to a boil.

Stirring constantly, boil for 4 minutes or until the mixture thickens.

Adjust the heat to low, partially cover the pan and simmer for 45 minutes or until thick and creamy.

Remove the pan from the heat, cover completely and let stand 5 minutes before serving.

Parmesan Walnut Linguine

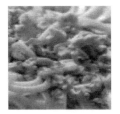

Ingredients:

8 oz linguine, uncooked

1/2 C walnuts, chopped

1/2 C almonds, chopped

2 garlic cloves, minced

1 tbsp extra virgin olive oil

1 tsp dried basil

1/2 tsp sea salt

1/4 C Parmesan cheese, grated

Directions:

Cook the linguine according to the package directions.

Drain well, rinse with cold water and drain again.

Place the walnuts, almonds and garlic into a bowl.

Sprinkle with the basil, salt and cheese.

Drizzle the olive oil over the mixture and toss gently to coat.

Stir the nut mixture into the linguine and serve immediately.

Basil Pesto Fettuccine

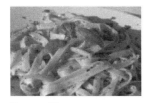

Ingredients:

2 garlic cloves

3 basil sprigs

1 tbsp pine nuts

1/8 tsp salt

1 tsp olive oil

2 tbsp grated Romano cheese

2 tbsp grated Parmesan cheese

10 C of water

1 large potato, peeled and diced

1/2 lb fresh green string beans

1 tbsp salt

1 lb. fettuccine noodles, uncooked

Directions:

Place the garlic cloves into the blender and mince.

Add the basil, pine nuts and salt.

Process until well combined.

With the blender running drizzle the oil into the blender and process until pureed.

Add in both types of cheese and blend until just mixed in.

If the pesto is too thick add a little water and pulse until you reached desired thickness.

Pour the water into a large saucepan.

Add the potato and beans and bring to boil, letting it boil for 10 minutes.

Stir in the fettuccine and salt and cook until the fettuccine is tender about 10 minutes.

Drain the pasta mixture well and top with the pesto sauce before serving.

Lemon Zucchini

Ingredients:

1 tbsp olive oil

1 lb zucchini, sliced into 1/2 inch pieces

1 1/2 tbsp parsley, chopped

1 tbsp lemon juice

1/4 tsp pepper

Directions:

Pour the oil into a skillet and place over medium heat.

Add the zucchini and cook 2 minutes stirring often.

Reduce the heat to low and cover the skillet.

Continue cooking 4 minutes or until the zucchini is tender.

Transfer the zucchini to a bowl.

Add the parsley, lemon juice and pepper and toss to coat.

Balsamic Spinach with Nuts

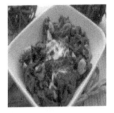

Ingredients:

2 tsp extra virgin olive oil

2 garlic cloves, minced

2 tbsp raisins

1 tbsp pine nuts

1 (10 oz) bag of fresh spinach

2 tsp balsamic vinegar

1/4 tsp salt

1/8 tsp pepper

1 tbsp Parmesan cheese, grated

Directions:

Pour the oil into a skillet and place over medium high heat.

Place the garlic, raisins and pine nuts into the skillet and stirring constantly cook 30 seconds or until fragrant.

Add the spinach and stirring constantly cook 3 minutes or just until the spinach is wilted.

Transfer the mixture to a serving bowl.

Pour the vinegar over the spinach, sprinkle with the salt and pepper and toss to coat well.

Top with the grated Parmesan cheese just before serving.

Cinnamon and Nut Topped Oranges

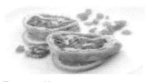

Ingredients:

1 tbsp sugar

1 tsp cinnamon

2 oranges cut in half

1/8 C walnuts, chopped

Cinnamon and Nut Topped Oranges

Directions:

Place the sugar into a small mixing bowl.

Add the cinnamon and stir until well combined.

Sprinkle the cinnamon sugar evenly over the oranges.

Top the oranges with chopped walnuts and serve.

Rose Apple Side Dish

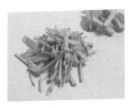

Ingredients:

3 sweet apples, peeled, seeds removed and sliced into sticks

2 tbsp sugar

2 tbsp lemon juice

1 tbsp rose water

1 dash of salt

Directions:

Place half of the apples into a blender

Sprinkle in the sugar.

Add the lemon juice and rose water.

Sprinkle in the salt

Cover the blender and blend 30 seconds or until coarsely chopped.

Add the remaining apples and blend another 20 seconds.

Pears in Pomegranate Sauce

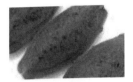

Ingredients:

4 ripe Bosc pears, quartered

1 1/2 C of pomegranate juice

1 C sweet dessert wine

Directions:

Place the pear quarters into a Dutch oven pan.

Pour the juice and wine over the pears and place the pan over medium high heat.

Bring the juice to a simmer then reduce the heat to low. Cover the pan and simmer 30 minutes, turning the pears over a couple of times during cooking.

Remove the pears with a slotted spoon and set aside.

Adjust the heat under the cooking juice to high.

Boil 10 minutes or until reduced to half.

Pour the juice over the pears before serving.

Herbed Rice and Brown Lentils

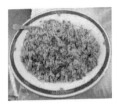

Ingredients:

1 C brown lentils, washed and drained

4 tbsp olive oil

1 C long grain rice

1 tbsp cumin

1 tsp salt

1/2 tsp turmeric

1/2 tsp pepper

1 1/2 C of warm water

Directions:

Place the lentils into a large saucepan and cover completely with water.

Place the saucepan over high heat and bring the water to a brisk boil.

Remove the pan from the heat, cover and let stand for 10 minutes.

Drain the lentils, rinse under cold water and drain again.

Pour the oil into a large pan and place over medium heat.

Stir the lentils and rice into the hot oil.

Stirring constantly cook for 2 minutes or until well coated.

Stir in the cumin, salt, turmeric and pepper well.

Pour the water into the pan and stirring constantly allow the water to come to a full boil.

Reduce the heat to low, cover the pan and cook 10 minutes or until all the water has evaporated.

Cornmeal Polenta

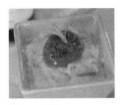

Ingredients:

6 C of cold water

1 1/3 C of cornmeal

1 tsp salt

Directions:

Pour the water into a saucepan and place the pan over medium high heat.

Stir in the cornmeal and salt and bring the mixture to a boil.

Stirring constantly, boil for 4 minutes or until the mixture thickens.

Adjust the heat to low, partially cover the pan and simmer for 45 minutes or until thick and creamy.

Remove the pan from the heat, cover completely and let stand 5 minutes before serving.

Parmesan Walnut Linguine

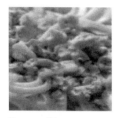

Ingredients:

8 oz linguine, uncooked

1/2 C walnuts, chopped

1/2 C almonds, chopped

2 garlic cloves, minced

1 tbsp extra virgin olive oil

1 tsp dried basil

1/2 tsp sea salt

1/4 C Parmesan cheese, grated

Directions:

Cook the linguine according to the package directions.

Drain well, rinse with cold water and drain again.

Place the walnuts, almonds and garlic into a bowl.

Sprinkle with the basil, salt and cheese.

Drizzle the olive oil over the mixture and toss gently to coat.

Stir the nut mixture into the linguine and serve immediately.

Basil Pesto Fettuccine

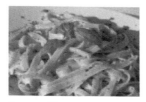

Ingredients:

2 garlic cloves

3 basil sprigs

1 tbsp pine nuts

1/8 tsp salt

1 tsp olive oil

2 tbsp grated Romano cheese

2 tbsp grated Parmesan cheese

10 C of water

1 large potato, peeled and diced

1/2 lb fresh green string beans

1 tbsp salt

1 lb. fettuccine noodles, uncooked

Directions:

Place the garlic cloves into the blender and mince.

Add the basil, pine nuts and salt.

Process until well combined.

With the blender running drizzle the oil into the blender and process until pureed.

Add in both types of cheese and blend until just mixed in.

If the pesto is too thick add a little water and pulse until you reached desired thickness.

Pour the water into a large saucepan.

Add the potato and beans and bring to boil, letting it boil for 10 minutes.

Stir in the fettuccine and salt and cook until the fettuccine is tender about 10 minutes.

Drain the pasta mixture well and top with the pesto sauce before serving.

Whole Wheat Eggplant Pizza

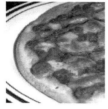

Ingredients:

2 tbsp olive oil, divided

1 small eggplant, cut into 1/2 inch slices

1 tsp salt, divided

1/2 tsp pepper, divided

1 C of tomatoes, seeds removed and chopped

2 oz feta cheese

4 tbsp fresh mint, chopped and divided

Directions:

Preheat one burner of a gas grill to high.

Place half of the oil into a mixing bowl.

Sprinkle the eggplant evenly with half of the salt and pepper.

Place the seasoned eggplant into the oil and toss to coat well.

Place the eggplant onto the grill and grill 8 minutes turning occasionally until tender.

Remove the eggplant and let cool enough to handle then chop into bite size pieces.

Pour the remaining oil into a bowl.

Add the eggplant pieces, tomato, cheese and half of the mint and toss to coat well.

Season the mixture with the remaining salt and pepper.

Place the pizza crust onto the grill and cook 1 minute or until grill marks are visible.

Remove the crust carefully.

Spread the eggplant mixture evenly over the crust.

Place the pizza back on the grill and close the lid and grill rotating 1/4 turn every 2 minutes.

Sprinkle the top evenly with the remaining mint before slicing.

Veggie Tortilla Wraps

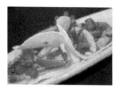

Ingredients:

3 tbsp extra virgin olive oil

1 tbsp red wine vinegar

1/4 tsp salt

1//8 tsp pepper

1 C plum tomatoes, chopped

1 C cucumbers, sliced

1 C green bell peppers, sliced

1/2 C red onion, chopped

1/2 C fresh parsley, chopped

1 C feta cheese, crumbled

8 (6 in) wheat tortillas

Directions:

In a small mixing bowl whisk together the oil, vinegar, salt and pepper until well blended.

In a large bowl toss together the tomatoes, cucumbers, bell pepper and onion.

Pour the dressing over the vegetables and toss to coat.

Add the parsley and cheese and toss again.

Fill one side of each tortilla with salad mixture and wrap with the other side.

Garlic Topped Spaghetti

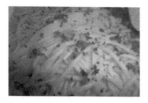

Ingredients:

1 (12 oz) box of spaghetti

1 stick of butter

3 garlic cloves, mashed

1 tbsp fresh parsley, chopped

Directions:

Cook the spaghetti as directed on the box.

Drain the spaghetti well and place in a serving bowl.

Place the butter in a skillet over medium high heat.

Cook the butter for 4 minutes or until it turns a golden brown.

Stir in the mashed garlic and cook 1 minutes or until fragrant.

Pour the mixture over the spaghetti and toss to coat.

Sprinkle with the parsley just before serving.

Toasted Hazelnut Cookies

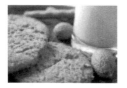

Ingredients:

2 C toasted hazelnuts

1 1/4 C sugar

4 egg whites

1/2 tsp salt

1 tsp vanilla extract

Directions:

Line 2 baking sheets with parchment paper and preheat the oven to 325 degrees.

Place the hazelnuts and sugar into the blender.

Pulse until very fine then remove to a bowl.

Place the egg whites and salt into a separate bowl.

Beat on high until stiff peaks form, about 5 minutes.

Fold the egg white mixture into the nut mixture.

Stir in the vanilla extract.

Drop the cookie batter by spoonfuls onto the prepared baking sheet.

Bake 15 minutes then rotate the pans on the racks.

Bake an additional 10 minutes or until lightly browned.

Cool the cookies completely on wire racks before storing.

Fruit and Nut Snack Mix

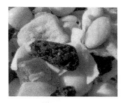

Ingredients:

1 1/2 oz toasted almonds

1 1/2 oz toasted hazelnuts

1 1/2 oz walnut pieces

1 oz. pine nuts

1 1/2 oz raisins

1 1/2 oz mixed dried fruit

Directions:

Place the almonds, hazelnuts, walnuts and pine nuts into a bowl and toss to combine.

Add the raisins and mixed dried fruit and toss again.

Store the snack mix in an airtight container.

Eggplant and Cheese Dip

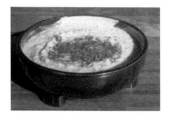

Ingredients:

1 (1 lb) eggplant

2 tbsp lemon juice

1/4 C of extra virgin olive oil

1/2 C feta cheese, crumbled

1/2 C red onion, minced

1 red pepper, seeds removed and chopped fine

1 jalapeno pepper, seeds removed and minced

2 tbsp fresh basil, chopped

1/4 tsp cayenne pepper

1/4 tsp salt

1 tbsp fresh parsley, chopped

Directions:

Preheat the broiler and line a baking sheet with foil.

Poke holes in the eggplant to allow the steam to release and place on the prepared baking sheet.

Broil 6 inches from the heat source for 15 minutes, turning every 5 minutes, until the outside is charred and the eggplant is tender with poked with knife.

Remove the eggplant and allow cooling enough to cut.

Pour the lemon juice into a large bowl.

Cut the eggplant in half and scrape the flesh into the bowl with the lemon juice.

Stir to coat the eggplant well.

Pour the oil into the bowl and stir until the oil is completely soaked into the eggplant flesh.

Saucy Apricot Pudding Cake

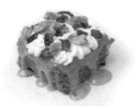

Ingredients:

1 C orange juice

1 C of water

1/2 C dried apricots

1/3 C + 1 tbsp sugar, divided

1 tsp orange zest

1/2 C of bulgur

2 large eggs, separated

2/3 C + 1/2 C low fat milk, divided

2 tbsp brown sugar

1/2 C walnuts, coarsely chopped

1 large egg yolk, lightly beaten

Directions:

Pour the orange juice and water into a saucepan.

Add the apricots, 1/3 C of sugar and orange zest.

Place over high heat and stirring constantly bring to a boil.

Reduce the heat to low and stirring occasionally cook 10 minutes or until the apricots are tender.

Stir in the bulgur, adjust the heat back to high and bring back to a brisk boil.

Reduce the heat and stirring occasionally cook 20 minutes or until the mixture looks like oatmeal.

Remove the pan from the heat and let stand 10 minutes, uncovered.

Preheat to the oven to 350 degrees and lightly spray an 8 inch baking pan with cooking spray.

Whisk 2 egg yolks and 2/3 C of milk together in a bowl. Slowly add the mixture to the bulgur and whisk until well blended.

Place the egg whites in a bowl and beat with a mixer about 5 minutes or until stiff peaks form.

Stir the egg whites into the bulgur.

Spoon the batter into the prepared baking pan.

Sift the brown sugar over the top of the batter.

Place the baking pan into a larger roasting pan.

Add enough water to the roasting pan to come about halfway up the baking pan.

Bake 35 minutes or until the cake puffs and is a golden brown.

Place one inch of water into the bottom of a double boiler and place over low heat.

Bring the water to a simmer.

Whisk the remaining milk, egg yolk and sugar together in the top of the double boiler.

Place over the simmering water.

Stirring constantly and adjusting the heat if necessary to keep a constant simmer, cook 5 minutes or the mixture is thick enough to coat the back of spoon and reaches 160 degrees on an instant read thermometer.

Quickly pour the sauce through a sieve into a bowl.

Cover and refrigerate 1 hour or until chilled.

Top the cake with the sauce and sprinkle with the walnuts.

Saucy Apricot Pudding Cake

Baked Cherry Pudding

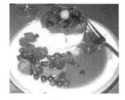

Ingredients:
1 lb tart cherries, pitted
1/3 C + 1/4 C sugar, divided
2 large eggs
2 tbsp flour
1 1/2 tsp vanilla
1/3 C of non fat evaporated milk
Assorted berries to garnish

Directions:

Preheat the oven to 375 degrees and lightly spray a shallow baking dish with a non stick cooking spray.

Place the cherries in a bowl, sprinkle with the 1/3 C of sugar and stir until well coated.

Spread the cherries evenly over the bottom of the prepared baking dish.

Bake 20 minutes or until the cherries are juicy and tender.

Break the eggs into a bowl and add the flour, vanilla and remaining sugar.

Whisk the mixture until well blended and smooth.

Pour in the evaporated milk and whisk until well blended.

Drain the juice from the baked cherries into a separate bowl and set aside.

Return the cherries to the baking dish and pour the egg milk mixture over the top.

Bake 12 minutes or until the pudding is set and slightly puffed.

Remove and pour the reserved cherry juice over the top.

Garnish with mixed berries before serving.

Baked Yogurt Cheesecake

Ingredients:

15 Melba toast

1/3 C walnut halves

2 tbsp extra virgin olive oil

1 C + 2 tbsp sugar, divided

2 (8 oz) pkg low fat cream cheese

2 1/2 C non or low fat Greek yogurt

7 egg whites

1 tsp cinnamon

Directions:

Preheat the oven to 325 degrees and fill a kettle with water to use as a water bath.

Spray a 10 inch spring form pan with cooking spray and wrap the bottom and sides with a double layer of aluminum foil.

Place the Melba toast and walnuts in the blender and process until it turns to fine crumbs.

Place the mixture into a mixing bowl and add the oil and 2 tbsp of sugar.

Toss the mixture until moistened through.

Press the crumb mixture into the bottom of the prepared pan.

Bake 10 minutes or until lightly browned.

Cool the crust to room temperature and leave the oven on.

Beat the cream cheese and the remaining sugar together in a mixing bowl until smooth.

Add the yogurt, egg whites and cinnamon and beat until well blended.

Spread the mixture over the cooled crust and place the spring form into a shallow roasting pan.

Add enough boiling water to the shallow pan to come up 1 inch on the spring form pan.

Bake 45 minutes or until set.

Lady Finger Trifle Dessert

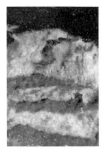

Ingredients:

60 lady fingers

1 C of water

4 tbsp brandy, divided

1 tbsp instant coffee granules

2 tbsp dried egg whites, reconstituted

3/4 C of sugar

1/4 tsp cream of tartar

1/2 mascarpone cheese

4 oz reduced fat cream cheese, room temperature

1 C chocolate shaving

Directions:

Preheat the oven to 350 degrees.

Place the lady fingers onto a baking sheet and toast 6 minutes or until just firm.

Remove and set aside.

Pour the water and 3 tbsp of brandy into a bowl.

Add the coffee granules and whisk until completely dissolved.

Brush the mixture over one side of each of the lady fingers.

Place one inch of water into a saucepan and place the pan over medium heat.

Place the dried egg whites, sugar and cream of tartar into a heat safe bowl that will fit just into the saucepan and place it in the saucepan over the simmering water.

Carefully beat the mixture on low speed for 4 minutes.

Adjust the speed to high and beat for 3 minutes.

Remove the bowl from the saucepan and continue to beat on high for 3 minutes or until fluffy.

Place the mascarpone and cream cheese into a bowl and beat until smooth.

Add 1 tbsp of the egg white mixture and the remaining brandy and beat until combined.

Add the remaining egg white mixture and stir until blended in well.

Place lady fingers in the bottom and up the sides of a trifle bowl.

Spoon one third of the cheese mixture over the top of the lady fingers in the bottom of the bowl.

Layer more ladyfingers over the mixture and add 1/3 more of the cheese mixture.

Layer more ladyfingers and the remaining 1/3 of the cheese mixture.

Cover and refrigerate at least 4 hours.

Sprinkle the chocolate shavings over the top just before serving.

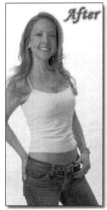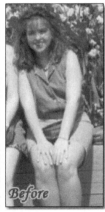

Recommended Reading: The Isabel De Los Rios Story

So...just who is Isabel De Los Rios?

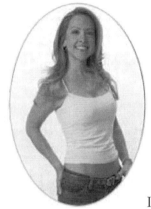

Isabel De Los Rios is a certified nutritionist and exercise specialist who has already helped over 25,000 people all over the world lose incredible amounts of weight, regain their health and permanently change their lives. She is the author of The Diet Solution Program and the Owner of New Body – Center for Fitness and Nutrition in New Jersey. She has become the #1 "go to girl" when it comes to Fat Burning Nutrition by several of the most popular fitness professionals around the globe. Isabel's cutting edge and completely different approach to nutrition is what sets her apart from all the rest. This approach has created results for so many once frustrated dieters. Her strategies work, hands down, as long as her simple principles are followed.

Isabel is able to educate clients and readers all over the world through her books, hundreds of online articles, seminars, and the media which all focus on the essential principles of fat loss nutrition and achieving a healthy, toned and vibrant body.

Isabel graduated from Rutgers University with a degree in exercise physiology (a pre-med curriculum). She is a Certified Strength and Conditioning Specialist, the highest and most advanced certification given by the National Strength and Conditioning Association. She is also a Holistic Nutrition Lifestyle Coach, certified by the Corrective Holistic Exercise Kinesiology (C.H.E.K.) Institute in San Diego, California. She counsels many special populations, including diabetics, heart disease patients, cancer survivors, and overweight individuals, as well as healthy individuals who wish to maintain health and prevent disease.

Isabel De Los Rios found her passion for nutrition as a teenager. The overweight daughter and granddaughter of type 2 diabetics, Isabel was told that she was doomed to suffer from the same health problems as the generations who preceded her. Not willing to sit around waiting for this grim prediction to become a reality, she pored over every nutrition and diet book available in search of the answers to her family's weight and health problems. This led her to personally seek out doctors and health professionals that were using nutrition to get great results (as far as health and weight loss) with their patients and clients.

She has since reached and maintained an ideal weight, is vibrantly healthy and shows no indication that conditions like diabetes will affect her as they have so many in her family. She truly enjoys a high level of wellbeing that not only surprises most people, but motivates them to achieve what Isabel has.

Find out more Today at:

http://tinyurl.com/paleodiets

Made in the USA
San Bernardino, CA
27 February 2013